Praise for *"Surprise I'm Still Here!!"*

". . . working through the mental and physical difficulties that come with this disease continues to be something that all myeloma patients and other cancer survivors face. I look forward to sharing this book with others."

Jack Aiello, myeloma patient

"A lovely and thorough "how to" book which gives the patient with newly diagnosed cancer, or even the patient who has had it for awhile, tips on dealing with the devastating diagnosis, the side-effects of therapy and the emotional stresses of such a life-changing experience. The author has opened her heart and clearly used her experiences to reach out and help others."

Jeffrey Wolf, MD, Director,
Myeloma Program,
University of California San Francisco

"Jane lives daily with something most of us hope we never have to—the diagnosis of a fatal, incurable disease. But this book is not about dying or about merely surviving. Jane's wisdom in her statement that 'only when Giving exceeds Taking is there Meaning in life' should enlighten all of us and show us a better path to enjoy life in all its fullness. It is her invitation to all of us to start living in whatever circumstances we find ourselves."

MarieAnn Thornburg, CEO, Posada Consulting

SURPRISE!
I'M STILL HERE!!

SURPRISE! I'M STILL HERE!!

Living with Incurable Cancer

Jane Rubey

To order additional copies of this book, contact:
Xlibris Corporation
1-888-795-4274
www.Xlibris.com
Orders@Xlibris.com
79356

Contents

Dedication

For Guido Tricot, MD, PHD, a preeminent researcher in the search for a cure for multiple myeloma. I am privileged to be in his care.

Dr. Tricot heads the Huntsman Bone Marrow Clinic at the University of Utah, Salt Lake City. *www.fightmyeloma.com*

Introduction

Recently diagnosed? Currently in treatment? In a relapse? In a remission? Wherever you are on this arc of dying, it is helpful to move past the fear and denial it generates. Only when we accept the inevitability of death can we fully appreciate the richness of life.

If you are living with incurable cancer, you are not alone. Though every situation and person are different, we all face related realities when we confront something larger than ourselves. It is my wish that you will find inspiration in these pages.

Remember, no one else can live your life. No one else is you. How you deal with the challenge of cancer defines a new you. I invite you to stop dying and start living. May you face this unique time in your life with hope and courage!

PART ONE

Opening

Knocked Down

Nothing can prepare you for those three dreaded words: "You have cancer." It can seem like the end of the world, especially if the diagnosis, as in my case, is for an incurable cancer such as multiple myeloma, bone marrow cancer. My life split in two parts: Before Cancer (BC) and After Diagnosis (AD). Life as I had known it was no more. I could no longer work. Play was limited by physical constraints and intermittent pain. My life would never be the same again. There is nothing quite like chronic cancer from which there is no vacation.

When you eat right and exercise seriously, you do not expect to fall into the deep hole that is cancer. But there it is. Bad things happen. You fall. After the dust clears and you look up to see if there is still daylight in your world, you can either give up and stay in your hole or climb out and make the most of the time you have left.

I was down but not out. I climbed out of that hole and am now faced with the reality of death.

I am dying!

Maybe not today, maybe not tomorrow, but the end is no longer out there in the vague future. At first, this wake-up call came as a brutal shock. But as time passes—it is now year 7 AD for me—I value every day as if it might be my last. When you have looked death in the eye, you are better able to see life. I try to live life to the fullest. I have no time to waste on trivialities; life is too valuable.

I often hear in my head, as I did when I was growing up, my mother's voice admonishing me, "Life is too short." Her caution to me has a different ring to it now that my days are numbered. A carefree youth can afford to squander some of life's precious moments. No longer. I have mastered the fine art of just saying, "No!" I avoid the worst of politicians, negative people, unsatisfying activities . . . . Of course, this streamlining of choices isn't limited to those of us with cancer; but I am amazed how it has helped me develop a laser-like sharpness for cutting through the dross in life, illuminating and concentrating on what's best.

Pick Yourself Up

Treatment felt like being hit with flying bricks from a building being destroyed by a tornado. When the winds calmed down, I was bruised and bloodied. It would have been easy to give up at that point and let the disease claim victory.

AD is where the tough get going. When things cannot get worse, you only have the choice of getting stronger.

In my treatment, an experimental protocol, I had two bone marrow transplants using my own adult stem cells. The procedure required that they hit me with enough chemo to kill my existing, cancerous bone marrow before infusing my own adult stem cells to build new, healthy bone marrow. In other words, the procedure has to come as close as it can to actually killing you in order to save you.

This is where the flying bricks came in. I could not dodge them. I needed to muster my wits and fight back.

Dust Yourself Off

As I lay waiting for my bone marrow to rebuild, I thought about what was most meaningful in my life. To keep me struggling to survive, I needed a vision to focus on. My most unshakable desire of that time was wanting to live to see my oldest grandchild, Megan, graduate from high school. She had just turned nine years old. Her two younger brothers, Spencer and Ashton, were seven and four; I didn't hold much hope of seeing them grow up. I thought if I could just hold on long enough to see Megan through grade school and high school, I would have grabbed the brass ring.

It's important to envision the future even though you cannot know how long it will last.

Today, Megan is sixteen and a blooming beauty! Hellooo . . . brass ring!!

Start All Over Again

So, here's the deal: stop dying and start living! Take it one day at a time. Easier said than done, of course, but cancer isn't for scaredy-cats. We must not cower in fear. We may not like the cards we are dealt, but we must play them to the best of our ability.

Cancer calls forth every bit of bravery we can muster. It uncovers inner resolve I did not know I had. At the end of each day, I can look back and say, proudly, "I did it. I survived another one." I am continually amazed by my own good fortune.

I recently ran into a friend I had not seen for a couple of years. She looked at me wide-eyed and remarked, "I thought you were dead!" I smiled as I exclaimed, "Surprise, I'm still here!!"

Before Cancer (BC)

Before I was diagnosed, I had been busy teaching nutrition and cooking. I was about to celebrate ten years of success with my website, *Nutritiously Gourmet*, which featured changing monthly menus and recipes that utilized sustainable, seasonal foods. My next step was going to be to publish a cookbook of recipes from my classes and *Nutritiously Gourmet.*

Family and friends knew me for my adherence to a healthy diet as well as extensive walking—not just short walks between the refrigerator and the stove, but daily circuits throughout the neighborhood and even lengthier hikes. Disease prevention was a major theme in my teaching, and I tried to practice what I preached.

My BC health, however, did not spare me from tripping over the brutal divide between BC and AD. I believe it did help me to weather the ferocious storm of chemotherapy and sustain my recovery, however. Eating right and exercising regularly have supported me through seven tough years, providing an unexpectedly high quality of life. I'm not just surviving—I'm living!

After Diagnosis (AD)

So, what does life AD look like?

It is time to unwind some of the wisdom gathered and recorded in your memories over a lifetime. Weave your past strengths into the life that cancer attempts to weaken. Here's a simple way to connect to inner power: Imagine starting at the end, the day you die, and working backwards through your life.

What do you want people to remember and say about you *after you are gone*?

What is unique about you that you want others to know?

What has been the meaning of your life?

As I consider how I want people to think of me, I return to a basic equation:

Giving - Taking = Living!

At different moments, some people are Givers and some are Takers. Some are both at the same time, giving with one hand while taking with the other.

We all know the Takers: people who shirk responsibility, who talk too much without saying anything, who look the other way when there is work to do, who are always nay-saying and negative. They drain the essence from life. When you are ill, Takers seem to threaten your very existence. You realize you are even more vulnerable AD than BC.

What and how you give speaks volumes about who you are. Givers are the people who are there for you, and you for them. When you are down but not yet out, Givers come by with fresh roses from their garden. They offer a steadying arm when crossing the street or climbing stairs. After one look at me, grocery baggers offer carry-out help.

More than ever, I am appreciative of the Givers. I am diligent with my smiles and thank yous, believing they inspire more good deeds. Love, generosity, and selflessness need to outweigh egotism, greed, and selfishness. We are all part of the Living equation.

I look for random acts of kindness that I can do to help push the Giving part of the equation. Giving can be difficult when you are sick, when you are so needy. Chemotherapy left me hairless, but I paid my hairdresser for one year of non-haircuts. He is also a cancer patient. It was important that I give him encouragement and that he be there for me when I regrew my hair. Thinking beyond myself and reaching out generates inner satisfaction and puts a smile on my soul.

So it's not surprising that I want to be remembered as someone who gave and, when given something, gave something back, as a person who knew that life is a gift and that love is life's beauty.

My low self-energy limits most of my volunteering for good causes, but I know that donations in kind or money are always welcome. Some days I get more phone calls and mail from solicitors for charities than I get from friends. Most of those requests are on behalf of giving organizations. The calls keep me in touch with the needs of the outside world and offer me an opportunity to give back.

Only when Giving exceeds Taking is there Meaning in life. That's another way of stating my equation. If you think about that equation, you'll likely find your life already has meaning. Living life is more than just surviving. Life is a gift. And the real meaning that defines life itself comes from love. Life without love is like a broken vase. It has no useful function; it holds no beauty. All that is best in the human experience stems from loving and being loved.

Love sustains our journey.

PART TWO

A Trio of Challenges

The Treatment Challenge

With the dreadful diagnosis still ringing in my ears, I was rushed to the hospital with failing kidneys. I couldn't feel my elevated blood calcium level, but it was pretty apparent that something was very wrong. My degenerated neck discs were supposedly unrelated. But as the evidence mounted, it was clear that I had multiple myeloma.

I began a two-year period of mistreatment at the hands of an oncologist who did not specialize in multiple myeloma. I slowly came to the realization that I was moving toward a dead end.

Since multiple myeloma is a complicated and relatively rare cancer, I realized that I needed to find doctors who specialize in my particular disease. I couldn't afford to keep wasting time with hit or miss approaches. I wanted the best treatment available. I needed an expert. I was open to something different, a new and possibly experimental approach. When you find yourself drinking from a glass that is already more than half empty, it is important that you pay attention to each remaining sip.

I had earlier used my computer to log onto the Internet to look up definitions of myeloma. Because I lived near world-famous hospitals, I assumed I would get the best treatment possible close to home. Yet soon, driven by desperation because of my failing treatment and body, I searched the Internet again.

I came to realize that, with perseverance, the Internet was a golden resource regarding treatments. Mostly by luck,

I happened onto the web site of the Myeloma Institute at the University of Arkansas for Medical Sciences in Little Rock (www.myeloma.uams.edu) which specializes in multiple myeloma. The Arkansas team is on top of current myeloma developments, and research protocols are available for cutting-edge treatments.

Traveling out of state for treatment takes serious commitment—an ability to pay the cost emotionally, physically, and financially. In my case, I would have to give up being near some of my regular and most important Givers—my children and grandchildren. That's partly why it can be tempting to seek out and settle for the easiest treatment plan. At least you're dying at, or close to, home.

Trying a novel treatment approach might pour some precious time back into my emptying hourglass. As I've mentioned, it's now 7 AD. While individual situations and responses vary a great deal, I am glad that I chose to undertake a rigorous treatment that offered the best long-term results with a high quality of life.

Let's get real: my treatment was grueling and gruesome, something only a desperate person would try. But the outcome five years later has been optimal, and I have years more, God willing.

So here is my challenge to you: Understand your disease and keep current with new developments, including opportunities for worthwhile and low-cost clinical trials. Near where you live or on the Internet, join a good local support group to educate and inspire you. When I see other myeloma patients who are doing well, I want to learn their secrets.

Symposia sponsored by the International Myeloma Foundation and the Multiple Myeloma Research Foundation are excellent sources of information. These resources offer good opportunities to locate the leaders in the field and identify other oncologists for second and third opinions regarding available treatments.

My current oncologist, Dr. Guido Tricot, moved from Arkansas to head the Huntsman Bone Marrow Clinic at the University of Utah in Salt Lake City (www.fightmyeloma.org). I find it impossible to separate the importance of the doctor from the treatment. Dr. Tricot has truly saved my life. It's your responsibility and challenge to find your own "life saver."

The Caregiver Challenge

Another essential member of your health team is your caregiver. Your challenge is to recognize who is the right caregiver for you, the person who is willing to share and understand your life-and-death decisions. This person may be your partner in life, a daughter or son, another family member, a good friend, or a counselor. You may have different caregivers who care for you in different ways—your physical, intellectual, and emotional needs—people who can go with you to the doctor, read the latest research news, help you strategize about treatments, and comfort you when the going is tough.

If your treatment or response or something else is not going well, you and your caregiver can find the courage to question and take charge. My husband, Chuck, never imagined that "in sickness and health" might lead to his being the major Giver in my life. On finding himself suddenly thrust into the demanding role of caregiver, he learned—along with me—to navigate the ins and outs of treatment. His ability to be flexible about his job and his willingness to accompany me halfway across the country to Arkansas, and now to Utah, helped save my life. I am forever grateful.

Here's a sweet example of Chuck's caregiving: At one point, I found it necessary to leave the hospital against medical advice. I was supposed to be discharged on a Friday, but a consulting doctor decided I should stay over the holiday weekend on starvation rations (Jell-O and popsicles—imagine!) just in case I developed an ulcer because of the wrong drug I had been given. I felt I could have died. Chuck and I said, "No way." He helped hold me up as we walked out of the hospital, no wheelchair offered because we had left against orders.

Living with someone who has cancer is not the same as living with cancer. Multiple myeloma can be quite crippling. Many vertebrae in my back have compressed with fractures, causing ongoing backache. I carry a pair of pillows to cushion hard seats. I try to keep the pain to myself as much as possible. It's part of my challenge to create a loving and playful space for me and my family.

The Safety Challenge

It is imperative to be careful. There are many ways you can meet the challenges of treatment and receiving care by paying attention to how, because of cancer, you are suddenly more vulnerable.

No matter how tired you are, consistently check the labels on IV bottles for the name of the drug you were told to expect and check a second time for the right dosage. Once during a hospitalization when staff tried to administer an anti-psychotic drug without my permission, I objected. My refusal didn't go over very well, but, hey, it is *my* body. Now, I diligently read all literature about the side effects of the drugs I take so I can better understand what my body is saying. And so I don't trip up—literally.

After a particularly grueling period of treatment, Chuck and I decided to celebrate with a cruise. During a stretch of rough seas, a woman passenger fell down the stairs and split her head open. The four doctors aboard were unable to do anything for her. I realize bad things can happen to anyone. I now hang onto all railings on stairs. I have no desire to end up like the unfortunate woman on the ship.

My willingness changed immediately about "watching my step," but it took longer to train my feet, which had a mind or mindlessness of their own and needed my coaching to move safely and surely in the right direction.

My neuro-*pathetic* feet have a tendency to trip me up with their lack of feeling. I also suffer from a built-in hazard, congenitally long feet. If your cancer eats your bones as mine does, it is not only important to stay upright, it is mandatory not to fall. I tested this dictum experientially, not once, not twice, but three times before it fully registered.

First Fall. The messiest time was in a parking lot while waiting for my husband to retrieve a coffee. My oncologist at the time—I have had four—suggested I do step exercises to build up muscle. Seeing a curb in front of the car and having some unscheduled time, I got out and managed a few ups and downs before losing my balance and toppling backwards onto the greasy asphalt, hitting my head and splitting my scalp. *Bang.* Think I banged some sense into my head about not falling? I did, but my feet needed more direction.

Second Slip-up. Another inelegant tumble took place in the hospital during one of the six one-week periods I spent getting chemo during year one, AD. One of the drugs in the chemo cocktail was very effective in wasting muscle. I grew progressively weaker and weaker.

In an effort to maintain as much strength as possible, Chuck would accompany me, along with my IV pole and walking sticks, as I ambulated through the hospital corridors. Observers suggested I might be ski conditioning. Yeah, sure. On one of these outings, the sticks and base of the pole had an argument, sending me sprawling onto the floor. I was stunned when I realized that the "Code Blue . . . Code Blue" coming over the intercom was about me. The resuscitation team descended rapidly and determined that I was in no immediate danger of departing this world. They hustled me back to bed, leaving me red-faced and none too eager to go for future walks.

Third Tumble. My last fall was at home in the patio. I went straight backwards onto the bricks, hitting my head. Since I was alone at the time, I tried to stop the bleeding as much as possible with my hand. I crawled across the patio into the house. By the time my husband got home, I had cleaned up most of the mess.

But that was it. No more. I cannot afford any more brain damage. I have had enough chemo to cripple my mental capacity as it is and leave me with a genuine case of "chemo brain." It took a while, but I met the safety challenge. Now I can say and mean and live with, "No more falls."

This safety challenge made me rise up and face an unpleasant fact of my disease. I must constantly be careful and vigilant.

Learn your own cancer challenges and rise to them. As the saying goes, "You have to fall to learn to walk." Practice until you get it right. In my case, the third time was the charm.

PART THREE

Rings of Freedom

Fresh Air

Meeting certain physical challenges, even emotional ones, can startle me into me a whoop of joy as I overcome another seemingly impossible roadblock that my cancer throws across my path. My determination and drive to battle those multiple myeloma challenges, at least to a truce, sometimes give me and my closest Givers an impossible gift. Imagine you're a kid and jumping rope without tripping, and then you're hovering, sort of flying, timeless, and you could do it forever.

One day I surprised my oncologist in Salt Lake City with an email in which I remarked that occasionally there are times when I forget I have multiple myeloma. These aren't long periods of time, not weeks or months, and sometimes only short moments. But they do give me the chance to feel alive again, to feel unburdened, unleashed, able to breathe freely.

It doesn't take long, of course, for the chronic backache or fatigue to bring me back to reality. But I look for small windows that I can open to allow fresh air to flow through into the stuffy room of my disease.

In talking with others about when the window appears and when the air flows in strong and fresh, I realize that I can have many more of those "feel-free" moments if I carefully listen to others with cancer and discover what stirs up their own sense of disease-free liberation. I only need to open my heart and imagine I'm catching a ride.

Similarly, I'm convinced that my own flashes of freedom can give others both hope and a way to escape the AD leash of disease, if only briefly. If lucky, those moments may stretch into a blissful interlude.

I have looked at my life AD and cataloged some of the brass rings I reach for while I'm on my myeloma merry-go-round. These rings of freedom shine with a bright luster. They form small windows through which flows refreshing air, a lightness where disease loses importance.

Each of the sections in Part Three can be such a window. They don't follow any particular order. Together, we can experience those people and special moments that are helping us to enjoy our final stage of life. Together, we can take hold of the dreams that are still possible. Use my special moments to springboard into your own special moments you can still seize. Share with others your rediscovered moments as the legacy, love, and grace you will leave behind when you are gone.

Children and Grandchildren

I live for my children, Margaret and Andrew. Not only are they great parents of my grandchildren, but they stepped up to the plate big time after I was diagnosed. Margaret set up what today would be called a blog for all interested parties to inform them of my progress during treatment. She was my voice when I couldn't even sit at a computer to send an email.

Andrew provided me endless recorded episodes of *Northern Exposure,* a TV serial about life in a rural Alaskan town. This TV distraction allowed me to mentally escape as I lay helpless on the couch, recovering from stem cell transplants. I can still see that moose walking down main street.

I am so lucky to have grandchildren. They are a major source of inspiration and joy for me. I have five altogether, three by Margaret and her husband Harrold, who live nearby, and two by Andrew and his wife Sheri, who are a day's drive away.

When Margaret's three children were very young, I took them to the mountains in the summers for an experience I called "Camp Cabin in the Woods." That was BC, of course, when I could take them swimming, hiking, picnicking—out into nature. We designed and painted a camp tee shirt each year, drew murals of our daily adventures, collected specimens of bugs and cones, raced twig boats downstream, panned for gold, went to the county fair, sang silly songs, and just did all those fun things together that campers do. I relive those joy-filled days through photos which, for me, open some favorite windows to let in the pine-scented air. I have yet to clean out my boxes of camp stuff—stickers, binoculars, bug boxes, whistles, fabric paints, books . . . it is hard to accept those days are over. And in fact, as I write about them, they are still very much alive.

My husband, Chuck, and I have invited each child when she or he turned twelve to join us on a trip to the national parks. We are especially fond of Yellowstone, the Grand Canyon, and Jackson National Parks. This has been a great way to spend special time with each child individually and share our love of nature and wildlife with them. The memories generated by these travels are more precious to me than gold or gems. Now Margaret's three are growing up, and I take equal pride in their school and sports achievements. Megan and Spencer are in high school, a dream I never imagined that I would live. And Ashton delights us with his love of baseball and nature.

I very much want to pass along to my grandchildren my passion about food and cooking. That's a tall order In today's nonstop round of sports and school activities, to say nothing of those incessant videogames I would rather forget. I do manage to carve out the time for a few junior cooking sessions. The Thanksgiving dinner that the grandchildren prepared from scratch was magnificent. They tirelessly scampered about the kitchen and lifted all the heavy pans and crockery I can no longer lift. I sat and watched and smiled (and gave a few suggestions) while the young cooks pulled off the entire feast by themselves, proving the adage, "It's not only food, but also hands that make the meal."

My children, their children, my grandchildren, all children—especially the little ones—work magic on me with the enthusiasm and innocence they show and give. When Andrew's boys, Aiden who is four and Liam who is two, come to visit, I find energy I didn't know I had. I love to watch them at play in a park or delighting at wonders of flowers and bugs that I would miss if not for them. Sitting in a grocery cart, they are high enough for eye contact. I can usually get a smile back when I send a wink or two. Their liveliness, rather than exhausting me, energizes me.

Talk about hope for the future; talk about feeling and living that hope. Small children everywhere embody and give you that hope.

Friends

It can be a major challenge to go from leading an independent life to depending on others. Both emotional as well as physical support take on a new level of importance. With energy always at a premium, fatigue lies ready to ambush. Having family and friends available to step in and help is essential. No longer can the basics of life—daily care, meal preparation, driving—be taken for granted. You need help.

Before I was Year One, AD, into this new life with cancer, I realized I needed more support than family and random friends offered. I selected twelve special "best" friends to be cheerleaders for me. I gave each an enameled wreath pendant that they can wear each December as a statement of friendship and support. Whenever I run into one of them when we are both wearing our necklaces, it is an indescribable moment of joy and solidarity for me. I am so blessed to have such friends. These Givers put a smile on my face and courage in my heart.

Weakened by illness, you appreciate the Givers in your life more than ever. You need to ask for assistance and find the humility to accept it with gratitude. Our thankfulness is part of the continuing equation of meaningful Living that puts Giving first, so that whatever Taking does subtract from Giving does not tire or weaken the lives of those giving friends around us.

Photos

Photos, especially in this digital age, have become a lifeline for me. I take more and more pictures to remind myself of the glorious life around me. It does not matter that I already have shelves full of albums. More albums just mean more events and scenery and people to look back over and relive. Photos are a wonderful way to enjoy the memories of life, both BC and AD. As an alley cat sings in the musical, *Cats*, "Let the memory live again."

Find a friend with a camera, or do it yourself. Capture those flashes of freedom as you grab life's brass ring. Are you bald from chemotherapy treatments? Take your photo with a hat, a bandana, or nothing—but wear a "thank-you-life" smile. Put it in your album next to the others, send your smile in a letter or email to your friends and family. That way, you keep the positive rumor mill going. Each photo says, "Surprise, I'm still here!"

Travel

I love to travel and share my stories. It is wondrous to experience other cultures and to imagine the challenges posed by climates and circumstances different from my own. I come home stretched and invigorated in body and soul.

My favorite BC trips involved walking and hiking. I became enamored of and proficient in using walking sticks. Now, AD, I carry them in the car in the event I encounter an uneven walking surface or stairs without a railing. Alas, no more Alps for these wobbly legs.

Today, Chuck and I favor sit-down travel where you stay somewhere for a week or use a ship as a moving hotel. I also substitute armchair travel for the actual thing. I belong to a travel group that meets monthly. Those eager beavers scour the earth to find interesting sights and experience exotic places. Their wonderful pictures and commentaries save me lots of time and money. I am also spared the exhaustion and jet lag. Not such a bad deal, really.

And for me, one of the best sit-down travel experiences possible is to go on a food and cooking expedition. A good food magazine or TV show can transport me on culinary adventures for several hours. My kitchen fantasies require neither money nor backaches nor tears from chopping onions. They contain absolutely no calories and, the best part, no cleanup afterward! As Julia used to say, *"Bon appétit!"*

New Threads

Initially, shortly after the AD era began, I hesitated to buy any new clothes. This is what I call "green banana thinking": Maybe I won't be around long enough for the bananas to ripen.

With my back fractured and shortened by several inches, I am no longer five foot ten. My old wardrobe no longer fits. Worse, all the organs that reside in my previously normal length torso are now squished forward into a belly bulge, something new to me. Not only does this expand my waist, but several fractured ribs stick out in front as well.

I often remind myself, especially looking at a smart outfit in a clothing store, that I am more than just my body. It's true that we need a body to be recognizable, but it exists primarily to house our souls. I am not willing to try living without my body any time soon, but it is my spiritual being that is the real me and keeps me focused.

To move forward and really live with this cancer, I have been forced to invest in some new clothes. In short, my BC wardrobe no longer works.

New duds, despite the crooked frame on which they now hang, are a definite morale booster. There are days when I get out of bed excited to wear something new. It helps put that smile on every morning. Hey, when you are really low, a little boost, wherever you can find it, goes a long way.

For someone frugal like me, I found it difficult to scrap perfectly good clothing. So you better believe I plan to stick around long enough to get my money's worth from this new wardrobe! And that's also my advice to you: try it on and see if it fits.

Wishful Thinking

It's fun to play "Make a Wish." This is not the same as make-believing "If I Won the Lottery." I'm talking about the kind of wishes that can be fulfilled and lived *n-o-w*, considering our physical and financial constraints.

Wishes offer a window to the future, hope for something special, and that brass ring of freedom. Wishes are a form of positive thinking, a means of reaching forward toward a desired goal. Even if a specific wish goes unfulfilled, your making it and dreaming of it a bit will boost your spirits and morale.

Some wishes of only a few words can take a long time to be fulfilled. "I wish I was stronger" has taken me several years of steady gym workouts to build back some of my devastated muscle. Other wishes can be both motivational and almost instantly gratified, especially now that it's AD. I sometimes make a deal with myself to motivate me to go to the gym. For example: "I would love to have a hot fudge sundae with coffee gelato and toasted almonds." This one works like the carrot dangled in front of the laggard donkey.

Here's my latest "wish upon a star." Last Christmas, my husband wanted to buy me a piece of jewelry. I said no, thinking, *I already have more jewelry than I can wear at any one time. Do I need more?* The real answer was no. But I still wished I had a little more.

So here's the solution that developed. I told Chuck: "I wish you would give me a thin, stacking ring to celebrate every five years of survival, AD."

My plan was to start with one now and wish for another on my tenth year anniversary of living AD. Maybe I can even score three! . . . or four!! before this is all over. It's that carrot in front of the donkey thing or, in this case, carats.

Make your wishful thinking work for you so you're not just lying on the couch dreaming about *what-if.* Use your wishes as incentives to keep thinking positively, eating right, and exercising.

The Blue Zone

One of the nicest things to happen to me shortly *after diagnosis* was when my daughter presented me with a blue handicap card. I didn't fully appreciate at the time what a fabulous privilege it would be to park inside the blue lines. It turns out to be worth its weight in gold, sort of a Medal of Freedom for the lame and faltering. Friends fight over me to be in their carpools. They covet their own blue card until I help them factor in what it takes to earn one—say, crippling cancer. I even feel a tiny bit warmhearted when paying taxes to a government that shows such commonsense compassion. Three cheers for the . . . blue!

Patience

It is helpful to practice patience. After all we are patients (wordplay intended). We need to relax and enjoy the journey. We will reach our destination soon enough. Our circumstances demand that we slow down, accept our limitations. We have no choice but to live with the situation as we find it. Impatiently trying to alter facts and reality just brings about frustration. I'm not suggesting that you give up and throw up your hands in defeat. But making the effort to make the most of a bad deal gives more pleasure than fighting continuously to defeat an unyielding monster. Patience, not anger, helps us as patients living with cancer.

Anticipation

Anticipation, not to be confused with impatience, is one of my favorite ways to add pizzazz to my days. I love to look forward to family celebrations. Birthdays are especially fun with the mystery of gifts and the promise of a slice of scrumptious cake. School reunions can build anticipation of seeing old friends and learning where they are on the path of life. I also like to anticipate visits from friends who come to stay a few days or who share a meal.

Don't be afraid to anticipate because you might suddenly have to cancel your plans. My husband and I support our local theater group and regional ballet. Having season tickets gives me excursions to look forward to, even if I have to miss out occasionally or leave at intermission.

Anticipation lets you begin to savor life's best moments even before you live them.

The Write Thing

Another way I keep connected and keep my focus forward is to write letters to the editor. At home, on trips, or waiting endless hours in waiting rooms, I enjoy keeping current with what's happening in the world by reading newsmagazines, and—would you guess?—food and travel magazines. When something rattles my cage or irritates me sufficiently to voice an opinion, I try to capture it in writing and submit a letter to the editor. Waiting the week or two it takes for turnaround is deliciously suspenseful. I never expect to see my letter in print, of course, but it has actually happened. Plus, I have the satisfaction of knowing that at least my opinions registered somewhere on someone before being rejected.

And a tip: Too tired to write or type? Some TV and radio news programs give out free 800-numbers so you can call in while the show is on (or later) and register your opinion about what you heard or saw. Instant polling is a boon to the bored.

Laughter

We all know laughter is the best medicine. You need to be able to laugh at yourself, at life, at cancer. And, oh yes, absolutely NO whining!

On a BC trip, we visited a monastery where the monks live in silence. Our tour leader—for some reason he was allowed to speak to us—told us they had a rule, "No murmuring." It seemed peculiar to admonish silent monks against murmuring, but I guess it shows the power of the tendency to mumble and grumble. I find the rule useful for myself. I have gained nothing from self-pity. No matter how bad things are—and I, for sure, know they can get seriously bad—the worst that can happen is that I die. Likewise, the worst thing that can happen to you is . . . you die. Simple. If you aren't ready to die, get on with the business of living! Make it the easy choice it is. When things seem unbearable, it is time to give up—right? *Wrong!* Fight!

It is too easy to give up. It takes real courage to fight, to go on. Smiling, not softly grumbling to yourself, helps.

To smile often, a sense of humor comes in handy. You may not be good at telling jokes or being funny ha-ha, but you can let yourself see the absurdity of situations, even your own. Laughing at yourself provides good release and relief. Finding the joke in something unpleasant, like a hairless head, enables you to let your irritation go away more readily.

Don't add to the misery of your disease. Blaming is not healthy. Grumbling is a waste of time. Constantly mumbling complaints is exhausting to you and others who are ready to be Givers. Living AD, we are already weakened and do not need to create unnecessary burdens.

Lighten up with laughter!

Simplicity

Cleaning out stuff helps to simplify life. One thing an unexpected fork in the road of life seems to do, especially when the new direction appears shorter than the original, is to make us more aware of stuff cluttering our lives.

I guess it is similar to moving to a new place, when people have to sort their stuff and decide what to pack and take and what to price for the garage sale. It seems some people who move actually throw away things they no longer want or need. Doing this used to be a foreign concept to me. Why would anyone want to get rid of something that is perfectly good and may have proved useful in the past? You might want it later on.

Well, let me tell you, cleaning out and clearing out stuff can be good for the soul. I use the excuse that I do not want my children to be left with the chore of sorting through my stuff after I am gone. Oh, sure. I am careful to save old baby pictures and news clippings of accomplishments, award certificates, and favorite rocks collected over time. It's important to me to leave traces of who I was in my lifetime in case the grandchildren ask for hard evidence or need to resurrect a favorite old recipe. But my file cabinets full of teaching notes and visual aids have been emptied, their contents recycled.

For a little fresh air and space, books can also be dusted off and moved out. I'm actually glad I saved favorite reads across the years. I love to read. When I could do little else AD, I reread many of my saved treasures. I then kissed them goodbye and gave them away to book friends or the library. My bookshelves are now cleared, the books having been liberated for others to enjoy. I, too, have been liberated.

Of course, there are books, and then there are *cookbooks*. My cookbook collection is a different story. I read cookbooks like another person reads mystery thrillers. I recently handed off close to fifty classics and nearly-new volumes to a charity fundraiser.

I still have a long way to go, but most drawers are cleaned out. Holiday decorations and ornaments have been distributed between my daughter and son. Photos have been sorted, albumed, and labeled. They will be easy to distribute or discard, in accord with my family's wishes. Now comes the difficult part:

Rule 1: Be careful not to refill cleared-out space.
Rule 2: Have a talk with the Givers of gifts. Incoming gifts need to be edible, such as chocolate or cheeses; use-uppable, such as candles; or something that can be returned to sender upon my demise, such as needlepoint pillows or the cozy lap robe that I recently received.

Clutter weighs down the soul. There is something liberating about less. Instead of feeling deprived, I feel enriched, even invigorated, after paring down. The freeing result: People are more important than things. Time seems more available. Shopping becomes more like an art tour. If I succumb to a purchase, it should be a gift for someone else.

Make no mistake; there are still closets and cupboards awaiting the sweep of my hand. Sorry, kids, you deserve a little fun. Secretly, I fear completing the job. It would then seem as if my "to do" list suddenly had nothing on it. That would be the real end of life.

Virtual Shopping

Having spent a great deal of time and energy in past years trying to get my name removed from catalog mailing lists in the hope of saving countless trees, I have finally given up. I have come to the frightening realization that I actually enjoy flipping the pages of catalogs.

A good catalog offers a delightful means of escape when you can no longer physically traipse the sidewalks and browse the shops in search of a needed gift or special toy for a grandchild. I love to sit back in my recliner and escape my AD reality with favorite catalogs. I thumb through listings of museum treasures, clothing, accessories, household décor, kitchen gadgetry, garden tools, trips to take, books—you name it, there are catalogs for everything, fantasies galore. The trick is not to succumb to their silent sales pitches. Remember: no more stuff. But looks are free, and pseudo-shopping has a very low energy requirement.

Note: Some people get the same pleasure and "no-buy" fantasies by browsing web pages or watching the shopping networks.

Pep

When in doubt (or just tired), nap. Napping is good. I have become quite addicted to my afternoon nap. It helps with my fatigue syndrome. In the evening, I can usually manage to prepare a simple dinner, eat, and watch some news before a postprandial nap sets in. I am careful not to let this cut into my sleeping time, which I also value highly.

The energy or peppiness thing is a tough one. My monthly blood work consistently comes up short in red blood cells (RBCs). Neither diet nor exercise seems to bump the number up to normal. A positive mindset is not a help. Oh, I know, it's the hemoglobin—the red pigment that shows the total amount of oxygen carried around your body—that seems to matter the most. The amount of hemoglobin is what the doctors watch. Fortunately, that value for me is now normal.

But I want more red blood cells. It's a weird number thing about something that seems real. With more on-the-page RBCs, I think I would have more energy. One month, the red blood cell count did register above normal. While it could have been a lab mistake, maybe it was the caffeine I drank that morning. I rarely drink caffeine, but that morning I had a double shot of espresso. Of course, unused to caffeine, it gave me a real jolt. In subsequent months, I tried to repeat my increased red blood cell count to no avail. I can get a burst of energy from caffeine, but it doesn't last. It is not a real solution to fatigue, though I seem to have enough pep to say a few more things about handling fatigue.

First, don't confuse fatigue with tiredness. Although related, tiredness results from activity. When I have a busy day, usually including exercise, I am tired by the end of it. I sleep really well. Regular exercise is essential for building strength and maintaining a healthy body. My oncologist wants me to ride an exercycle twenty minutes daily. I figure if I ride the elliptical for thirty minutes four or five times a week, plus use a few other strength-building machines at the gym, I satisfy his prescription. Best of all, it makes me feel good.

Second, scheduling is important. I find one activity a day works best for me. I sometimes manage a simple errand in addition to my regular exercise. My husband takes care of many errands, often known as chores, like food shopping. Chuck has learned the difference between cilantro and Italian parsley, how to find a good melon (ask the produce person), and the importance of organic foods, especially strawberries. I love to go to the market, but it exhausts me. If I do the farmers' market plus some cooking, I have exhausted my daily activity allowance.

Nighttime outings are tough to think about scheduling and tougher on my body when I do. Chuck and I sometimes leave theater events at intermission. I am glad my book club switched to afternoon meetings. We cancer types aren't the only ones getting "older" and wanting to relax with our feet up in the evenings.

I also try to schedule "down days." I intentionally do not fill in every box on my calendar. I leave one empty every three or four days. Sometimes, even that day will get filled, but it must be something very important. I value my "down time."

Third and still important, don't overdo it. Avoid exhaustion, which is the state of *over*tiredness. Exhaustion can wear you down and jeopardize your immunity. When you start flagging, slow down and take my prescription: a refreshing nap.

De-Stressing

Not every day is a delight. There are those blue, even black, days. Everyone has ups and downs. Sometimes the despair can seem overwhelming. I try to keep it at arm's length rather than giving in to it. It helps to distract myself with an activity such as a good drama on TV that engages more positive emotions. Downs are followed by ups; that is how we know they are downs. Here are some of my thoughts about handling distress and de-stressing.

Celebrate. The nicest thing happened to me Month One, AD: I celebrated my sixty-fifth birthday, and I got Medicare! I wouldn't be here today without Medicare. And now, with the advent of health care reform, may our country's health system offer better solutions for all cancer patients!

Write about it? Some reputable self-help books say that a good way to dispel anger and to integrate the wholeness of the maddening cancer experience is to write about it and then tear it up. Throughout my treatment days, people often asked if I was keeping a journal. (I wasn't.)

I found it a slow slog, plodding forward on nerve-dead feet, slumping from back pain, fatigued from missing red blood cells (and lack of hemoglobin). One day, out of curiosity, I started to list my cancer/drug/radiation-induced side effects. When I had filled a page full of ailments and still hadn't finished, I stopped writing. Quickly, I tore up the sheet. I didn't want what I had written to define me. No one really wants to know the awful details. That is for me, alone, to know. I don't want pity. I don't want to grumble or even whine. I want to live and be loved for that real me inside, not my broken body. I did not want to remember the details of those ordeals.

You don't need to finish what you're writing before you tear it up. Don't write yourself into box.

Say thanks. I do, however, find one kind of writing always to be positive. I keep a Gratitude Journal. Each day I try to note three things for which I am thankful. In this way, I regularly take a few moments to count my blessings.

Don't be shy about crying. Crying can be especially relaxing and de-stressing. I cry easily, sometimes for joy, sometimes for sorrow. It may be easier for women to cry than for men, but I recommend it to everyone.

I remember one time when my eyes just found themselves dripping. It was when I was being a good person and contributing to research for a cure to multiple myeloma. Since my cancer involves the bone marrow, researchers love to collect samples of bone and marrow for their studies. One guy, a torturer disguised as a kind Southern gentleman, would extract from me nine—count 'em, nine!—bone marrow biopsies in a row. Patients become resigned to one or two over a year because of checkups. But nine at once is really cruel. The second time this happened to me, someone in the next room who was having one single bone marrow biopsy was screaming. Needless to say, I needed to cry a bit.

Quiet Time

I have never mastered meditation, when you empty your mind and find absolute peace. New research tells us that a blank mind consumes twenty times as much energy as a conscious mind. It appears that "doing nothing" is really "doing a lot."

I do find, however, that sitting quietly is restorative. Daily, I put my feet up and attempt to do nothing. (Well, sometimes I drift into a nap.) This appearance of "doing nothing" is a newly learned behavior for me, having spent a lifetime keeping super busy. Let's face it: I now have the luxury of "wasting" time. I no longer feel guilty about this. I am off the frenetic treadmill of life.

Open Windows

When things look dark, remember it takes light to cast shadow. You may have to think halfway around the world to find the day of your night, but it is there if you look on the bright side. I find reading helpful. It transports me. I get to visit other places, meet new people, stand in their shoes for awhile. Sometimes their troubles make mine look smaller.

When your world seems to crash down around your feet—think diagnosis, treatment, bad lab results—it is time to open a window and escape to a different world. It could just as easily be art or music, but I find solace in the natural world. I love seeing animals, especially wild animals. When I can't go in person, I travel through photographs. *Nature's Best,* a quarterly magazine, collects the most magnificent pictures of animals and natural beauty I have ever seen. I keep all the back issues nearby, enabling me to escape my current world if it suddenly turns dark. Because I have enjoyed seeing the wonders of our National Parks and viewing many fantastic animals in the wild, I can use my imagination to combine my experiences with the photographs and enjoy the beauties of nature as if I were actually there in person.

You have many windows you can open, some in your own home. I am lucky to be asked to dog-sit. My daughter, Margaret, has a white fluff ball named Lucy that brings boundless energy and affection when she visits. Lucy loves to take us walking. She also is happy to snooze quietly in my lap. Either way, Lucy exudes unconditional love.

Perhaps the most therapeutic ongoing source of life at our house is bird watching. Chuck and I have put up two feeders; each appeals to different species of birds. We have binoculars and an identification book close at hand to distinguish the varieties.

We never cease to be awed by the tremendous activity and energy of the little song birds. It inspires us to watch them feed and fly fearlessly. They appear so fragile yet seem to confront their world with pluck and bravado. They offer a rich example of what it means to be alive and sing about it.

Ultimately, nothing sings "life" louder than springtime. Spring is my favorite season. If I am lucky, bulbs that I have forgotten burst from the earth and decorate the garden. My greatest love is the flowering trees. I just planted another crabapple; that makes four now. I have fruitless cherries and a plum as well. I sometimes think I would love to cut their branches of blooms and bring them inside, but they are a perfect work of art as they grow.

Remember, you can have open windows all around you and without risking chill drafts.

Surround yourself with things of beauty: family photos, fresh flowers, artistic wall decorations, garden annuals, lighted candles—whatever it is that gives your life a boost. I am passionate about natural minerals such as crystals of quartz or chunks of malachite. It amazes me to feel a slab of petrified wood or the weight of natural copper or of a piece of meteorite. Minerals that catch the light, such as labradorite, ammonite, or quartz, are my favorites.

Also, surround yourself with voices that speak of life. I am lucky enough to have inherited a great grandfather clock. He announces time in a deep, resonant voice. I set my other clocks so each one tells the time at a slightly different moment. That way, I can hear each one call out the time in their own voice. When I get up in the night, I often know what time it is without looking at a clock. When sleepless, I have a friend in the night.

My Favorite List

I love lists. In no special order, here is a list of a few suggestions for living with cancer:

- Get a good recliner
- Stand up slowly
- Count your blessings daily
- Be courageous
- Look people in the eye and smile
- Smile when you're alone
- Eat chocolate
- Look for luck
- Love a dog
- Hang a bird feeder
- Love your family
- Tell your loved ones you love them
- Eat more chocolate
- Ask for help when needed
- Drink water, lots of it
- No whining
- Laugh and cry
- Pick up your feet when you walk
- No more stuff
- Practice patience
- Wear your best clothes
- Be informed about your disease
- Enjoy good music

Bottom Line

Love those whom you hold dear, whether near or far.
This love is the source of joy and the essence of life.

PART FOUR

Closing

Last Chance

Sometimes we put off doing things we find difficult or may even dread, such as repairing a torn relationship or apologizing for a mistake. We may feel guilty or sad because of some hasty action, even one long ago. Before checking out of AD, it's a good time to clean the slate. Yes, it is difficult to ask for forgiveness. Yes, it may seem easier to let a wound fester rather than take our medicine and begin a healing process. Yet wholeness is not possible as long as there are rifts in our life.

I was recently given an opportunity to apologize for a mistake from my past. It was a big deal for me; I hadn't seen this person since graduation, fifty years ago. When I mentioned the incident and asked her forgiveness, she brushed it off as if it were a minor offense. I knew, however, that she remembered the incident, and it must have also gnawed at her. The result for me has been a feeling of relief and deep serenity. Asking and receiving forgiveness is deeply satisfying. When your days seem numbered, it is a good time to make amends and create positive memories for everyone in your life.

The saying, "one foot in the grave," suggests the second foot is due to follow any moment because you are near death and the gravedigger stands shovel-ready. I, for one, am not interested in thinking that way. Even if others see my fellow cancer survivors and me as having one foot in the grave, we really have the other foot free, with which to dance. True, we need to revise our dance routines a bit. Perhaps the Hop or

One-Step is more our style. Anyway, cue the music—loud but not too fast. And if we join hands or dance with a supportive partner, we might even make it through the entire tune!

I recently saw the movie *This Is It.* The documentary captures the "King of Pop," Michael Jackson, rehearsing for an upcoming tour. The young people Michael chooses to dance with him are also filmed expressing their joy and ecstasy at just being on the same stage with him. After more than an hour of magical song and dance, Michael seems pleased with the rehearsals and declares, "This is It."

His prophetic words echo what we now know; he gave it his best for the last time. His example provides inspiration for those of us living with cancer. We can live to the fullest and then, when "this is it" for us, we can put away our dancing shoes, knowing that we have done our very best, and quietly slip away.

Dear Friends, we have our work cut out for us. We have come to the last hurrah. We have no time to lose and no time for rest. We must remain ever vigilant to swat away any negative distractions. Now is our time to show just what we are made of and to be our very best. So let's get on with it. Let's open up the doors and windows of our minds and hearts and . . .

Celebrate Life!

Acknowledgments

Heartfelt thanks go to Fran Ryan who insisted I do this; George Truett, beloved friend and copyeditor *extraordinaire*; early readers and encouragers: Guido Tricot, MD, Anne Hamilton, Mary Louise Armsby, Diane Benson, Gloria Flynn, Carolee Houser, Marge Johnson, Marge Moser, Dede Muhler, Sharon Salomon, Barb Schumacher, and Sue Studier; and, of course, to my wonderful family for helping me hang in there. A portion of the proceeds from this book is being donated to myeloma research.

Some Useful Resources

American Cancer Society (ACS): *www.cancer.org*

Clinical Trials: *www.clinicaltrials.gov*

Handicapped Card: *http://arthritis.about.com/od/driving/a/ handicappedparking.htm*

International Myeloma Foundation (IMF): *www.myeloma.org*

Leukemia and Lymphoma Society (LLS): *www.Lls.org*

Multiple Myeloma Research Foundation (MMRF): *www. themmrf.org*

University of Arkansas, Myeloma Institute for Research and Therapy: *www.myeloma.uams.edu*

University of Utah, Huntsman Cancer Institute: *www. fightmyeloma.org*

Note: The Arkansas and Utah clinics do transplants on an outpatient basis, saving lots of money as well as allowing patients and their caregivers a more comfortable living situation.

Made in the USA
Lexington, KY
18 August 2010